SIMPLE HERBAL & AROMATHERAPY RECIPES FOR YOUR BODY, MIND & SOUL

SIMPLE HERBAL & AROMATHERAPY RECIPES FOR YOUR BODY, MIND & SOUL

ESTELLE CARRAZ, C.M.T, N.D

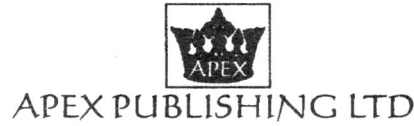

APEX PUBLISHING LTD

First published in 2004, Updated and reprinted in 2008 by
Apex Publishing Ltd
PO Box 7086, Clacton on Sea, Essex, CO15 5WN, England

www.apexpublishing.co.uk

Copyright © 2004-2008 by Estelle Carraz
The author has asserted her moral rights

British Library Cataloguing-in-Publication Data
A catalogue record for this book
is available from the British Library

ISBN 1-904444-07-5   978-1-904444-07-7

All rights reserved. This book is sold subject to the condition, that no part of this book is to be reproduced, in any shape or form. Or by way of trade, stored in a retrieval system or transmitted in any form or by any means, electronic, mechanical, photocopying, recording, be lent, re-sold, hired out or otherwise circulated in any form of binding or cover other than that in which it is published and without a similar condition, including this condition being imposed on the subsequent purchaser, without prior permission of the copyright holder.

Typeset in 12pt Baskerville

Cover Design Estelle Carraz

Printed and bound in Great Britain

Herbology

Natural and herbal remedies have gained enormous popularity over the last 30 years. However, many cultures, including early American settlers, have used the earth's natural resources to treat, cure and alleviate a variety of ailments for generations.
Herbology is the study of plants and their healing properties. There are several types of herbology systems used today, they include: Chinese, Ayurveda, Western, Native American and European. Despite their terminology and varying types of herbs, they all use natural resources, plants, roots, leaves, flowers and bark to promote health and well being.
The common methods for preparing herbs are pastes, juices, powders, poultices, salves, teas, whole herbs, extracts, pills, infusions, syrups and ointments. The method chosen for preparing herbs and herbal remedies is closely related to the symptoms of the specific ailment that is to be treated. Each method used for preparing herbs can provide different healing components. For this reason, one herb can be used to treat a variety of ailments. Plants have been used internally and externally to prevent and rejuvenate the body's system for centuries. The medicinal use of plants can be extracted from flowers, stems, seeds, leaves, roots and bark. The knowledge of these plants and what effect they may have upon the body is the practice of herbology.

Where do you get all your loose herbs and natural products?
At your nearest health stores, I recommend 100% organic products.

Aromatherapy

For centuries, many cultures have used exotic aromas ceremoniously. Recently, it has been discovered that aromas play a significant role in our overall health. Like many alternative health therapies, aromatherapy has rooted itself in mainstream popular culture over the last 40 years. As more information becomes available and more people learn about the benefits of aromatherapy, it becomes increasingly popular. Aromatherapy uses aromatic essential oils to improve the body's physical and emotional health. Essential oils are known as the "life force" of plants: They are highly concentrated, volatile oils, extracted from herbs, flowers, leaves, resin, bark, fruit rinds and roots.

When inhaled, the brain (lymphoid system) channels the effects of the oils throughout the body, balancing your body's system. Essential oils may also be absorbed by the skin and carried throughout the body via the circulatory system to reach internal organs. (Note that many essential oils must be diluted before applying them directly to the skin.)

If you have never experienced aromatherapy and essential oils, you may want to visit a Certified Aromatherapist or Massage Therapist that uses the oils, or if you prefer to dabble in aromatherapy on your own, make sure to dilute the concentrated oils with a base oil so as not to overwhelm yourself. This is especially important for small children or individuals with sensitive skin.

Where do you buy your pure essential aromatherapy oils?
At your nearest health store, find one that resonates with you! I recommend that the oils are 100% pure.

Massage Therapy

The interest in massage therapy has steadily increased in the last 20 years. A healing art that's been around since ancient times, massage therapy offers an unlimited number of benefits that can touch each person individually.
Massage therapy provides numerous therapeutic benefits for health, fitness and mental well-being. Massage helps improve the body's circulation, increases blood and lymph flow, stimulates the nervous system and affects internal organs as well as all the muscles. Massage therapy is a healing art that encompasses the manipulation of soft tissues, positively affecting and improving health and well-being. There are many styles of massage, including: Acupressure, Reflexology, Swedish, Deep Tissue, Lymphatic drainage and more.
Because there are so many different styles of massage it's important to find the massage therapist that offers the style that best fits your needs, in order for you to get the most from your session. Massage therapy can relieve muscle tension, strain, soreness and strain as well as insomnia, arthritis, bursitis, headaches, digestive problems, stress, anxiety, depression and much more. Not only does massage feel good, but helps to improve your range of motion and relax your muscles, it can also enhance your overall health and well-being.
Therapeutic massage may not be appropriate for some individuals. It is always important to consult with your

doctor before you receive a massage, especially for those individuals with infectious diseases, skin problems, imflammation of the veins, and cardiac conditions.

Make sure your massage therapist is certified.

Healthy, Beautiful Skin

Taking care of your skin has never been more important than it is today. Daily exposure to toxins, pollutants and chemicals affect our skin, that's why it is important protecting it from the harmful effects of the environment. Taking good care of your skin starts from the inside. Proper nutrition, diet and supplementation can help make your skin healthier. Cleansing and moisturising your skin daily protects it from exposure of toxic elements. Beginning a daily internal and external regimen will give you a jump-start in having healthier skin that looks and feels great.
As we age, we start to notice fine lines in our skin. To help keep your skin looking youthful, you could begin a daily regimen that exfoliates and nourishes the skin. This special treatment should contain naturally occurring alpha and beta hydroxy acids, that penetrate deep into the skin's layers to stimulate the cell's renewal process. Lactic acid, fruit acids and other natural alpha hydroxy acids are combined with beta hydroxy salicylic acid and natural herbs for sustained, long-lasting action. Other natural soothing and nourishing herbs for the skin include green tea, hyssop, calendula and chamomile. They will exfoliate your skin without damaging it and will help to reduce the appearance of fine lines, wrinkles and other visable signs of aging. Taking care of your skin today will prove beneficial in the future.

All natural beauty products can be found at your health store.

Recipe for Eye Makeup Remover
(Grandmas recipe from the past)

This recipe will take you seconds. All it takes is a trip to your refrigerator and a jar of mayonnaise. Scoop a little into a smaller jar and then use as required. Apply gently using fingertip and remove with a wet cotton ball. Refrigerate remaining mayonnaise.

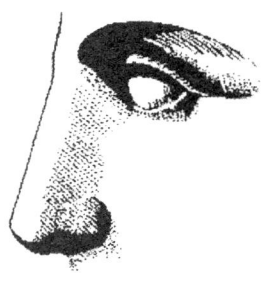

Tea Tree Mouth Wash

Use as a general mouth wash to combat infections and icky bad breath.

Ingredients:
5 to 6 drops of tea tree oil
Glass of warm water

Add your 6 drops of tea tree to a glass of warm water
Mix well
Rinse the mouth
Gargle once or twice daily, after brushing teeth.

Herbal Beauty Recipe

Facial masks are beneficial for removing dead skin, unclogging pores and helping prevent premature lines and wrinkles. Applying a facial mask once a week can dramatically improve your skin's overall health.
If you're interested in making your own facial mask with ingredients you can find in your refrigerator, check out the two facial mask recipes. These masks will leave your skin feeling soft and smooth and looking great!

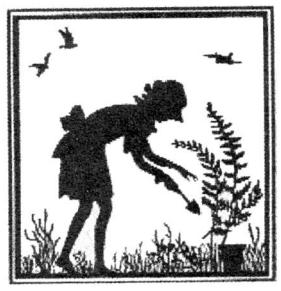

Cucumber Avocado Facial Mask
You will feel as cool as a cucumber

Ingredients:
1/2 cup chopped cucumber
1/2 cup chopped avocado
1 egg white
2tsp. powdered milk

In a blender combine all of the ingredients until they form a smooth, paste-like consistency. You can apply the mask immediately to your face and neck in a circular upward motions, or refrigerate it for 30 minutes.
Leave the mask on for 30 minutes, or until dry. To remove the mask simply rinse your face and neck with warm water, followed by a cold rinse. Finally, pat dry your face and neck.

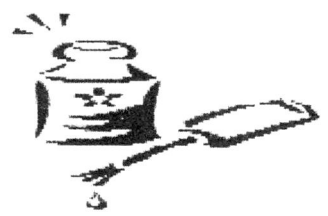

Earth Mask Recipe

Get back to earth and feel it's energy

Ingredients:
1 cup of dirt (any kind)
1 cup of water
3 Teaspoons of milk (Skim or 2%)
1 tbsp of sour cream

Mix dirt and water into a liquid paste. Then add the milk and sour cream. Apply to face. Leave on until dry. Then wash off with warm water.

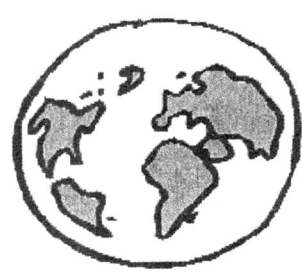

Bubbly Bubble Bath
Lots of fun & bubbles here...

Ingredients:
2 cups of soap flakes or grated soap
1 gallon water
1/4 - 1/2 cup glycerin
2 cups shampoo
Scented oil of your choice

Mix the soap flakes, water and 2 tbsp glycerin in a pot and set over low heat, stirring ocasionally until the soap has dissolved. (This liquid soap can be stored in a covered container and used as an all-purpose soap or hand soap in the kitchen.) In a bowl, add 2 cups of this mixture to the rest of the glycerin, shampoo and add a few drops of your scented oil. Put into a quart container and store covered at room temperature. When you're ready to bathe, add about one cup to your tub as it's filling.

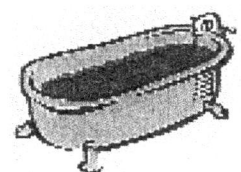

Zesty Lemon Mask
A refreshing and tightening face lift!

Ingredients:
Juice from half a lemon, strained
1 egg white

Beat together the egg white and lemon juice for three full minutes. Apply directly to your face avoiding your eyes, and leave on for 30 minutes. After 30 minutes, rinse your face with warm water and apply a moisturizer or cream.

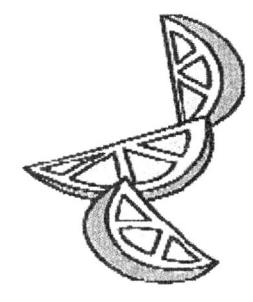

Cleopatra's Ginger Honey & Milk Bath

Relax like a Queen in this luxurious bath

Ingredients:
6 drops off essential ginger oil
1/4 cup honey
1/4 cup whole milk

Add ingredients to hot bath water. Soak!

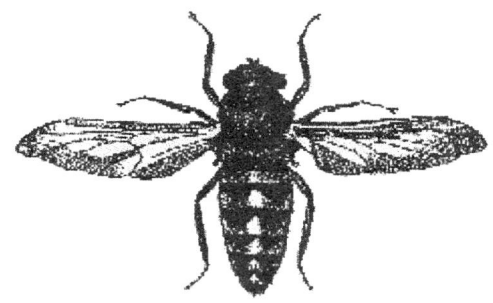

Vanilla Lip Gloss
Yummy kissable lips

Ingredients:
1 Tablespoon Petroleum Jelly
1 Tablespoon Aloe Vera Gel
1 1/2 teaspoons Coconut Oil
1/2 teaspoon Vanilla

Heat ingredients together in a double-boiler and pour into jars. Cool and seal.
Dab your lips! Kissable and yummy.

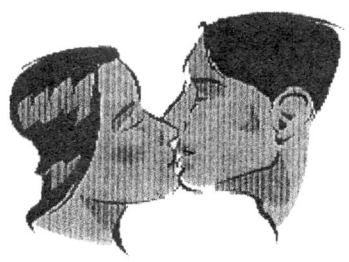

Make Your Own Hair Gel

Flax seed is so good for you that you should go out today and buy yourself a bag. It is one of the richest sources of Omega-3 fatty acids which aids in lowering high blood pressure cholesterol and triglycerides levels by as much as 25 and 65 percent. This prevents blood clots from blocking arteries which is a really good thing, obviously as we grow older, but did you know that by just adding a little water bringing it to a boil and allowing it to cool, you will find yourself a great hair gel. Try 2 Tablespoons of flax seed along with 1 cup of water. Bring it to a boil and then allow to set for about 1/2 hour. Strain and when it has completely cooled, add a drop or two of lavender oil (or your favorite scent) and then transfer to a clean wide mouthed jar with lid. Use as you would any hair gel product.

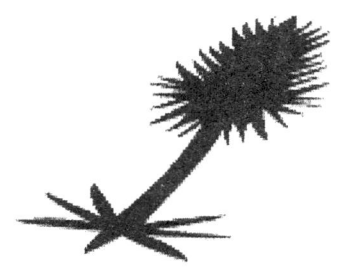

Honey Body Glow
A great way to invigorate your skin

Ingredients:
1 cup runny honey
1/2 cup of crushed sesame seeds
Sprinkle dried herbs: mint, lavender
1 pinch of cinnamon powder

Mix all ingredients in a bowl
Rub the thick goo all over your body
Wait for 1/2 hour then shower.

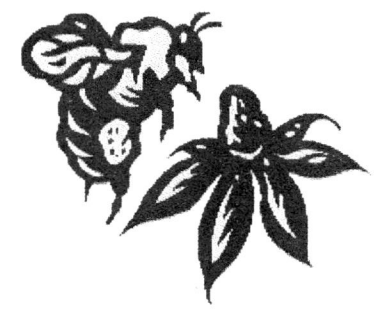

Yogurt Body Polish

Let your skin shine with this soft yogurt polish.

Ingredients:
2 tbsp finely ground rice
2 tsp turmeric powder
5 drops of sandalwood oil
2 drops of jasmine oil
Splash of water
2 cups of yogurt

Mix all ingredients in a bowl
Smear onto your body
Yogurt restores the natural pH of your skin and moisturizes it.

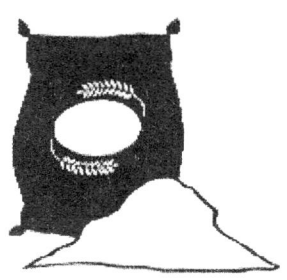

Cellulite Body Scrub

Let this mineral rich scrub seep into the skin to break down those fat cells.

Ingredients:
2 tbsp purifying mineral rich clay
2 tbsp sea salt
3 drops of nutmeg oil
3 drops of grapefruit oil
Water

Mix all together, adding a little water to make a light paste. Wipe vigorously over desired area of the skin. Once the paste is dry, rub the skin. Shower and apply some floral water spritzer.

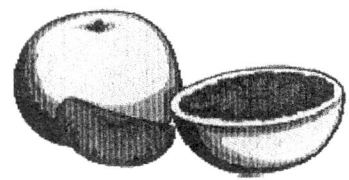

Carrot Face Puree

Ideal for overworked, mature , dry skin

Ingredients:
2lbs of carrots
1 tbsp of jojoba oil
5 drops of carrot oil
3 drops of orange oil
1 egg yolk

Puree all ingredients in a blender
Dab puree all over the face
Sit back and relax for 1/2 hour
Rinse off with cold water.

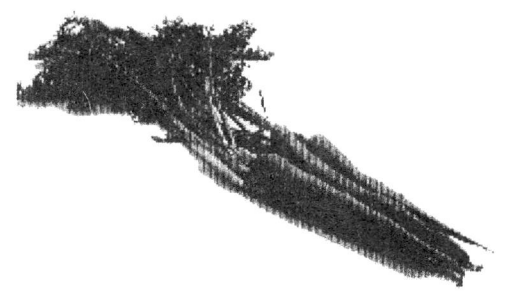

Juicy Lip Balm

Moisten thirsty lips with this yummy all natural lip balm.

Ingredients:
3/4 cup of cocoa butter
1/4 cup of jojoba oil
12 drops of sweet orange oil
5 drops of carrot oil
1 tsp of honey

Melt cocoa butter, jojoba oil and honey together
Remove from heat, add oils
Pour into a jar then cool it off
Dab on your lips.

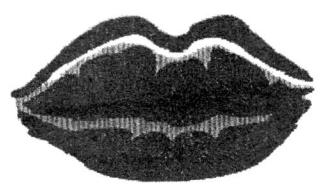

Shape Shifter Chest Salve

A wonderful chest salve to open the lungs, and inspire deep breathing. Wonderful for cold and flu symptoms

---

Ingredients:
3/4 cup cocoa butter
1/4 cup sweet almond oil
10 drops of eucalyptus oil
8 drops of peppermint oil
4 drops of lemon oil
4 drops of cajeput oil

Melt together cocoa butter and almond oil
Remove from heat, add all oils
Pour into a small jar and cool
Rub on chest area and inhale.

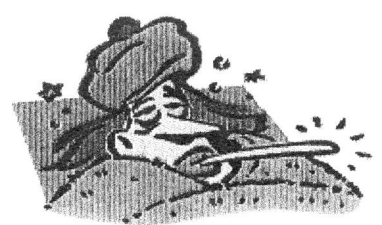

Foot Reviver

Exfoliation scrub for tired, achy or sore feet

Ingredients:
2 cups of fine sea salt
5 drops of tea tree oil
3 drops of peppermint
Sprinkle of lavender flowers
Dash of water

Make a fine paste
Rub the bottom of your feet
Massage them in a circular motion
Enjoy then rinse them off with hot water.

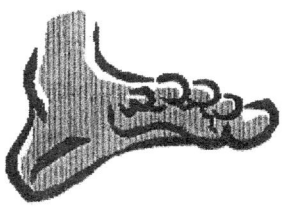

Euphoric Diffuser Salts
An instant pick-me-up anytime of the day

Ingredients:
1 cup of coarse sea salt
1 tbsp of crushed rosemary herb
1 tbsp of crushed lemongrass (fresh)
5 drops of lemongrass oil
5 drops of rosemary oil
3 drops of sweet orange oil

Combine all ingredients in a lidded jar.
Shake well, uncap and enjoy the aroma.

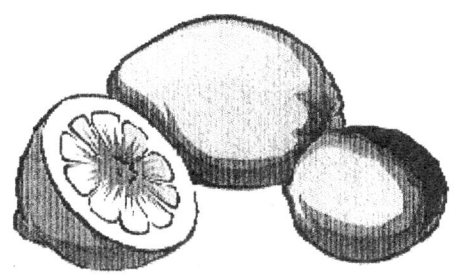

Floral Water Spritzer

A fragrant floral spritzer to soothe your soul.

Ingredients:
2 cups of distilled water
1 drop of lavender oil
3 drops of geranium oil
Handful of fragrant fresh rose petals

Put all ingredients in a bottle and shake vigorously
Let it sit in sun of 3 days
Strain the water and put into a spritzer bottle
Apply to face and body.

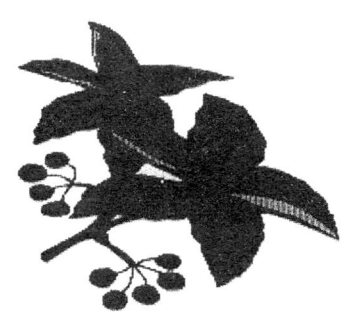

Exotic Scalp Treatment

For smooth silky soft hair.

Ingredients:
2 cups of coconut milk
3 drops of ylang-ylang oil
3 drops of jasmine oil

In a large bowl mix all ingredients and warm up
Apply to hair
Gently massage the scalp in a circular motion
Wrap a towel around the head
Let sit for 1/2 hour
Rinse thoroughly
And let hair dry naturally.

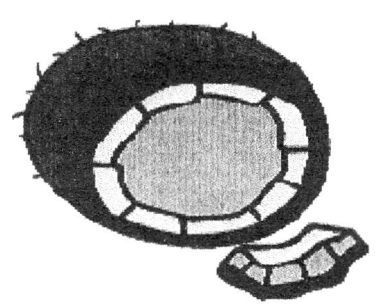

Synergy Massage Oils

The best way to absorb the therapeutic value of the oil is thru your skin.

Ingredients:
1 1/2 cup of almond oil
Euphoria: Lemongrass, lemon, sweet orange
Energy: Peppermint, rosemary
Zen: Clary sage, lavender
Prana: Eucalyptus, tea tree
Shape Shifter: Nutmeg, cinnamon
Mantra: Sandalwood, cedarwood
Eros: Patchouli, ylang-ylang
Flower Power: Rose, orange, lavender, lemongrass, and ylang-ylang

In a small bottle put 5 drops of each oil with your base almond oil
Shake well, and apply to your body.

Perfumed Oil Blendz

A long lasting aroma for the body. You will smell irresistible

---

Ingredients:
Blue skies: Blueberry, lavender, clary sage
Gaia: Sandalwood, carrot and patchouli
Harvest moon: Cinnamon, nutmeg, clove
Herbal lore: Lemongrass, thyme, sweet basil
Mystic Kiss: Ylang-ylang, vanilla, nutmeg
Razzle Dazzle: Raspberry, vanilla
Savannah: Gardenia, lemon, peach
Sweet Dreams: Jasmine, coconut oil, lavender, chamomile, ylang-ylang.

Fill a small aromatherapy bottle with a base of grapeseed oil
Add 6 drops of each oil
Shake well and apply to wrist and neck area.

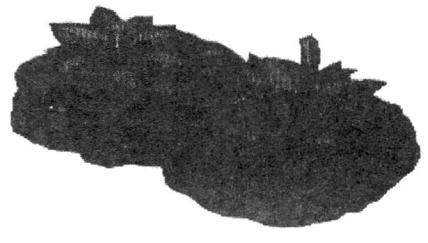

Lavender Soap Spheres
These delightful lavender soaps scent your skin for hours.

Ingredients:
4 ounce bar of castile soap
1/3 cup of water
40 drops of lavender oil
1/3 cup of dried lavender flowers

Cut the 4 ounce bar of castile soap into small cubes.
Place them in a heatproof nonmetallic container
Heat 1/3 cup of water until nearly boiling
Pour the hot water over the soap cubes.
Let it cool down a bit
Mix the soap and water with your hands
(if cubes float on top of water, add more soap)
Let the soap and water sit for 9 minutes until mushy
(reheat if necessary)]
While the soap is melting add 40 drops of the lavender oil
Add 1/3 cup of dried lavender flowers
Mix well with hands
Let it cool down
Separate soap mass into 4 parts
Form them into spheres
Place them on a 9" square piece of cotton cheesecloth
Gather cloth at top tightly and tie up
Hang spheres for 3 days until bone hard
Remove cheesecloth, and voila!
You can rewrap them in some real cool material & label them.

Pain Reliever For Toothache
As an emergency measure, to ease pain

Ingredients:
1 to 2 drops of Clove oil

Apply 1 to 2 drops of clove oil directly to tooth. Using your fingertip, gently massage into the area.

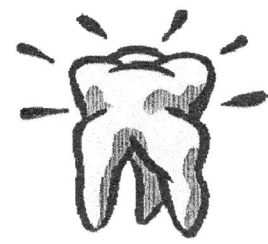

Cooler for Sun Burnt Skin

Let the heat escape from your skin with a cooling cucumber chamomile blend.

Ingredients:
4lb whole cucumber (whipped in blender)
1/2 cup of chamomile flowers
2 drops of lavender oil
2 drops of tea tree oil

Put all ingredients in a blender and whip it up.
Apply to sun burnt area
wrap in gauze and relax for about 30 minutes.

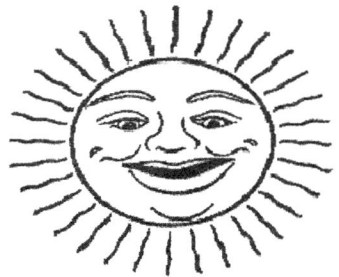

Aromatherapy Bath Oils

The bath is a perfect place to enjoy the sensual pleasures of aromatherapy oils.

Bath time blends:
For passion: Ylang-ylang, patchouli, sandalwood
For relaxation: Lavender, chamomile, clary sage.
For energy: Grapefruit, lemon, peppermint, pine
For immune boosting/respiration:
Rosemary, peppermint, eucalyptus.
For detoxifying: ginger, sage, rosemary

Mix 3 drops of each oil in your hot bath and enjoy the aromas!

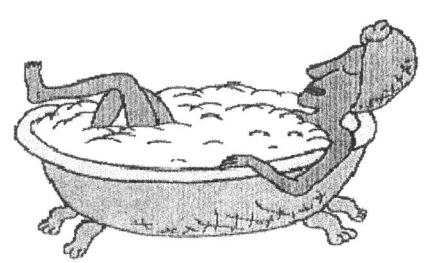

Edible Body Dust

This sweet sexy dust is great to feather over the body. For smooth silky skin

Ingredients:
1 cup of honey powder
Some feathers

So simple, just dab the soft feather in the powder
Brush over the body in a caressing stroke
Now use your imagination, it's edible!

Tea Tree Egg White Mask

Helps your skin draw out toxins. Cleanses and tightens up pores.

Ingredients:
1 egg
6 drops of tea tree oil

Break egg, separate the white from the yolk.
Add the tea tree oil.
Beat the white for one minute by hand
Apply to face and let it harden
Wash off with warm water
Pat dry.

Avocado Body Moisturizer

This thick avocado paste is wonderful for dry skin.

Ingredients:
3 whole avocados
1 tbsp of vitamin E oil
6 drops of sweet orange oil

Peel and pit the avocados
In a blender whip them up
Add your viatmin E oil and orange oil
When perfectly whipped - no lumps
Put in a bowl, scoop out applying it to desired body
Now take a hot shower
Your skin is moisturized and nourished.

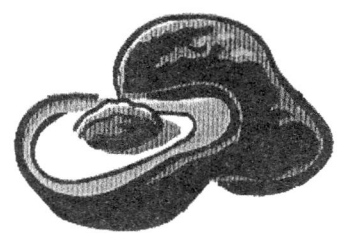

Lavender Facial Toner

This alcohol-free toner is great to clarify, brighten and cleanse your face.

Ingredients:
1 cup of witch hazel
6 drops of lavender oil

Pour the cup of whitch hazel in a bowl
Add 6 drops of lavender oil
stir it up
Using a cotton swab gently apply to face.

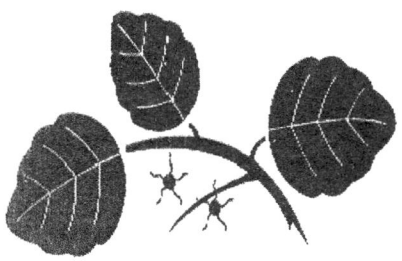

Oatmeal Facial Cleanser for Oily Skin

Oatmeal gently exfoliates the skin while absorbing excess oil.

Ingredients:
1 cup of oatmeal flour
6 drops of lemon oil
3 drops of peppermint oil
Water

In a bowl combine all ingredients
Add a little water until you get a light paste
Apply to face and gently massage
Leave on for 15 minutes
Rinse with cold water.

Anti-Wrinkle Eye Gel

This natural mild exfoliating gel works like alpha-hydroxy acid due to it's powerful enzymes.

Ingredients:
1 papaya fruit

Very simple, peel the papaya
mash them into a bowl
You should have a good goo
Apply around eyes
Relax and wait for 20 minutes
Wash off with lukewarm water.

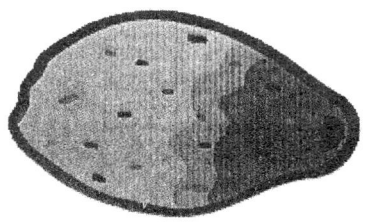

Natural Hair Helpers

Easy to make and simple to do recipes for all types of hair.

Ingredients:
Dry Hair: 10 drops of carrot oil,
1/2 cup of coconut oil
Thin Hair: 1 cup celery juice, 2 eggs,
10 drops of rosemary oil
Oily Hair: 1 cup of apple cider vinegar,
10 drops of lavender oil
Dandruff Hair: 10 drops of peppermint oil,
crushed mint leaves
Thick/Curly Hair: 1/2 cup of coconut milk,
10 drops of jasmine oil
Blond Hair: 1/2 cup of lemon juice,
10 drops of chamomile oil
Dark Hair: 1/2 cup of cocoa powder,
2 tsps of vanilla extract, 10 drops of clary sage
Red Hair: 1/2 cup of raspberry juice,
10 drops cinnamon oil

Whatever the ingredients are mix or blend them well together.
Apply to hair, gently massage the scalp.
Wait for 20 minutes, rinse well with hot water.

Quick Tips
For eyes, skin & face

Ingredients:
Tired eyes: 2 thin slices of cucumbers
Place them on your eyes to cool off
Oily dirty skin: salt & a drop of water
Mix and wipe face
Skin brightener: lemon juice use a cotton
ball and wipe face
Blemished skin: cut a fresh slice of pineapple
Wipe blemished area
Skin nourisher: 2 kiwis
Scoop out the middle and smear onto face.

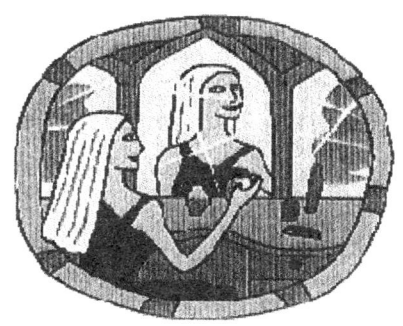

Peppermint Foot Powder
A minty fresh foot powder. Helps to keep them dry

Ingredients:
1 Cup of Baking Powder
1/2 cup of Baby Powder
6 drops of Peppermint oil

Mix all ingredients in a bowl
Massage powder onto feet
And Voila!

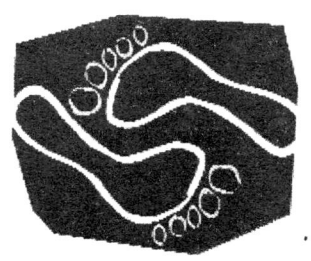

Aromatherapy Potpourri
A fragrant easy to make potpourri for anyplace

Ingredients:
3 cups of dried mini rose buds
2 cups of lavender flowers
1/2 cup of chamomile flowers
1/2 cup of dried lemon zest
10 drops of lavender oil
5 drops of rose oil
5 drops of sweet orange oil

In a large bowl mix all ingredients together
Place in small bowls around the house and enjoy.

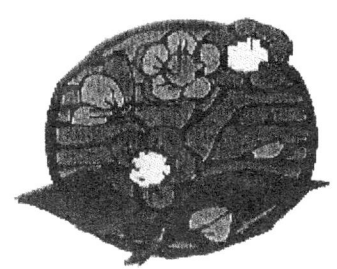